THIS IS A PERSON.

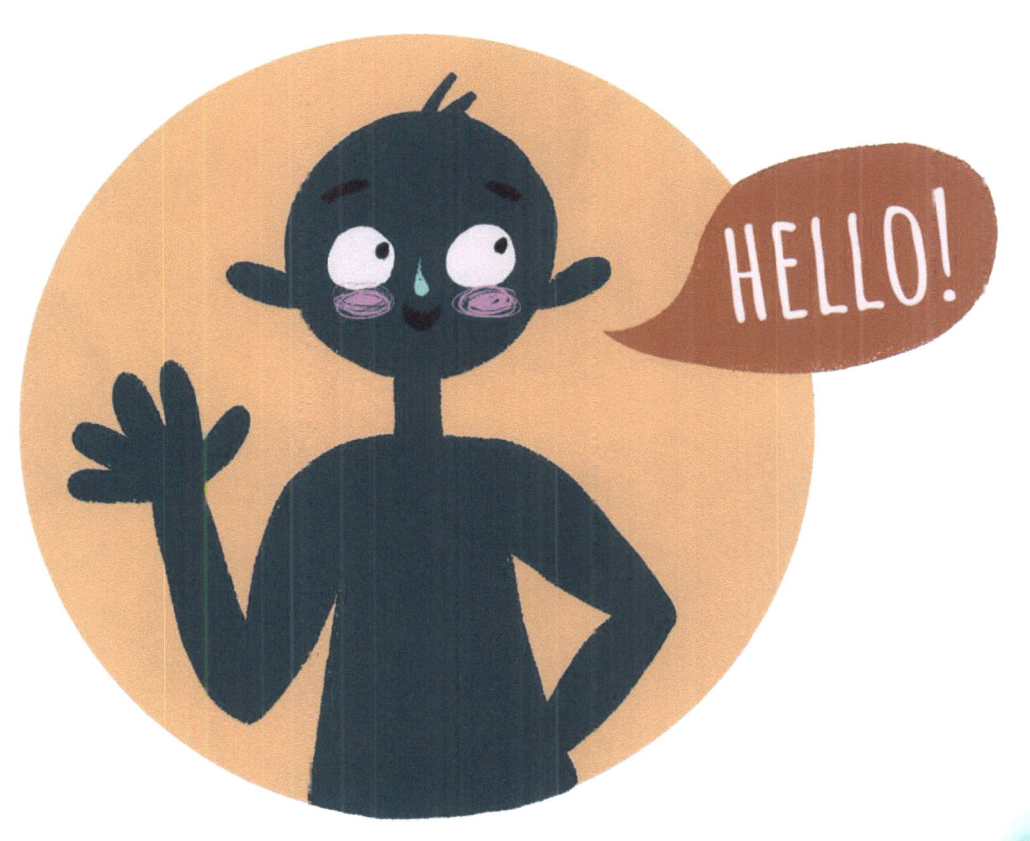

A GROUP OF MANY PEOPLE IS CALLED A POPULATION.

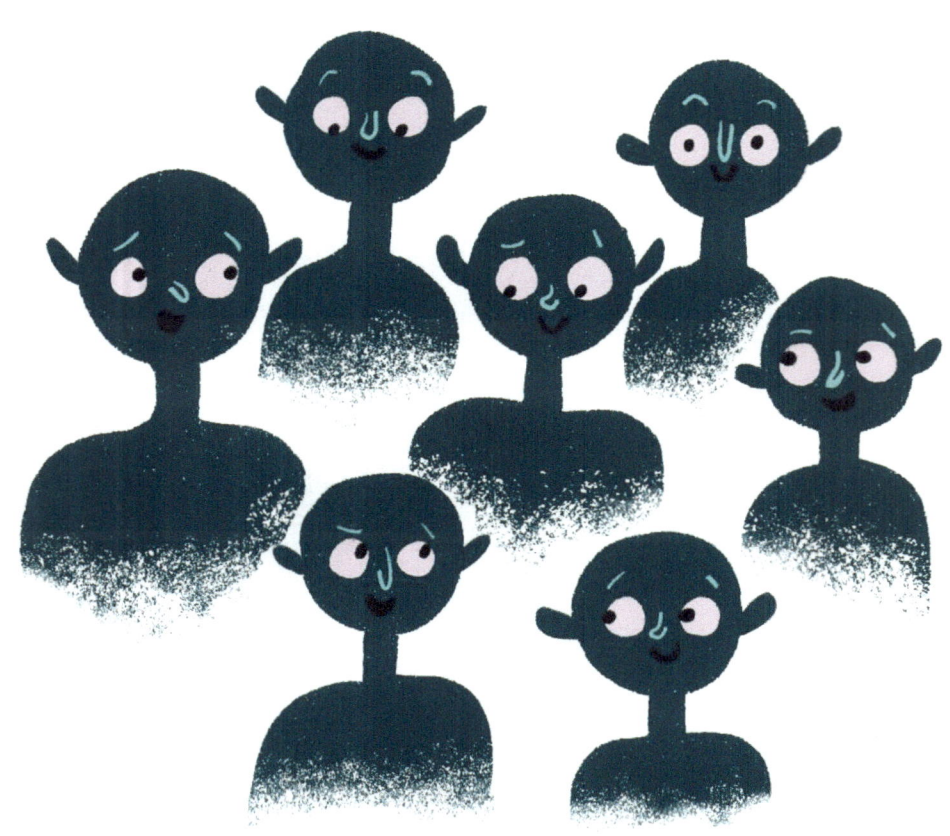

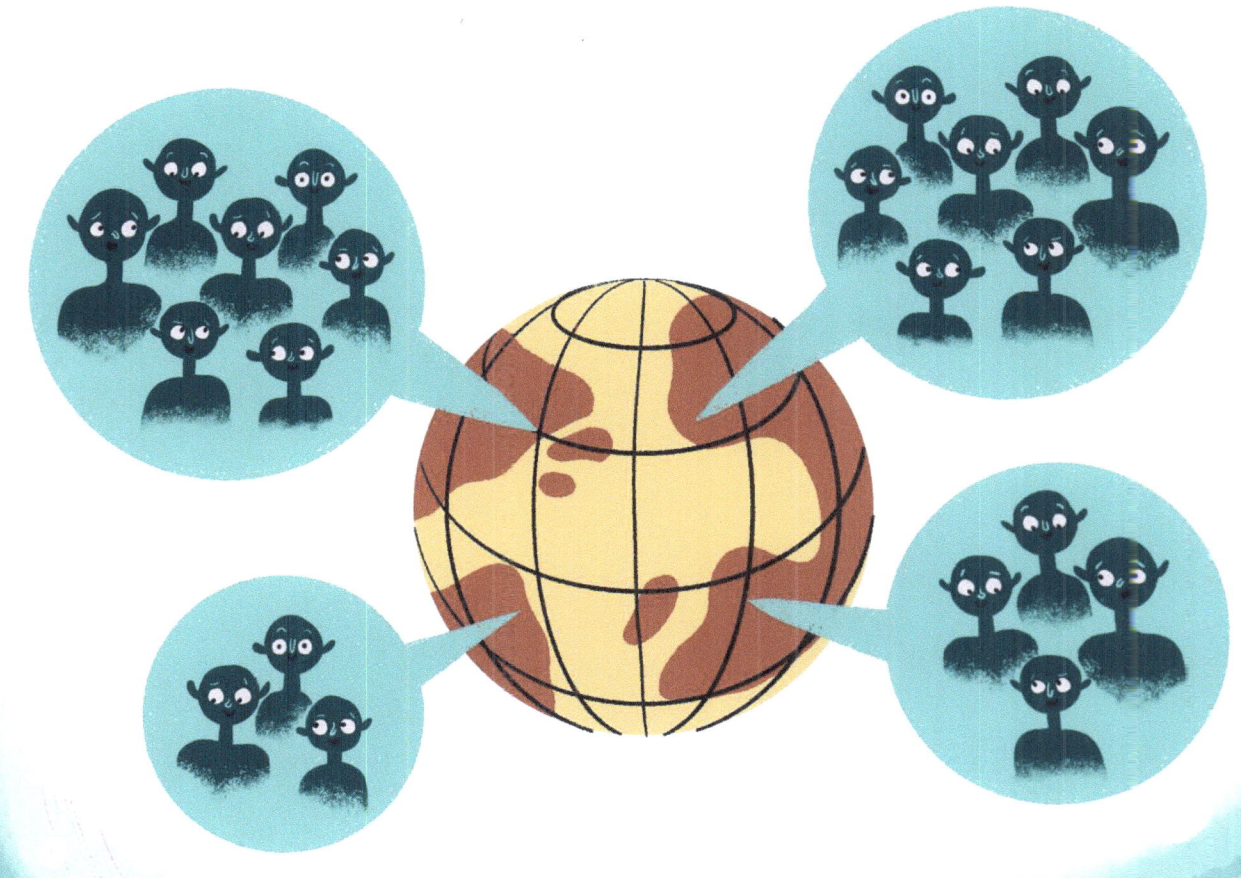

AND CAN BE ORGANIZED INTO GROUPS.

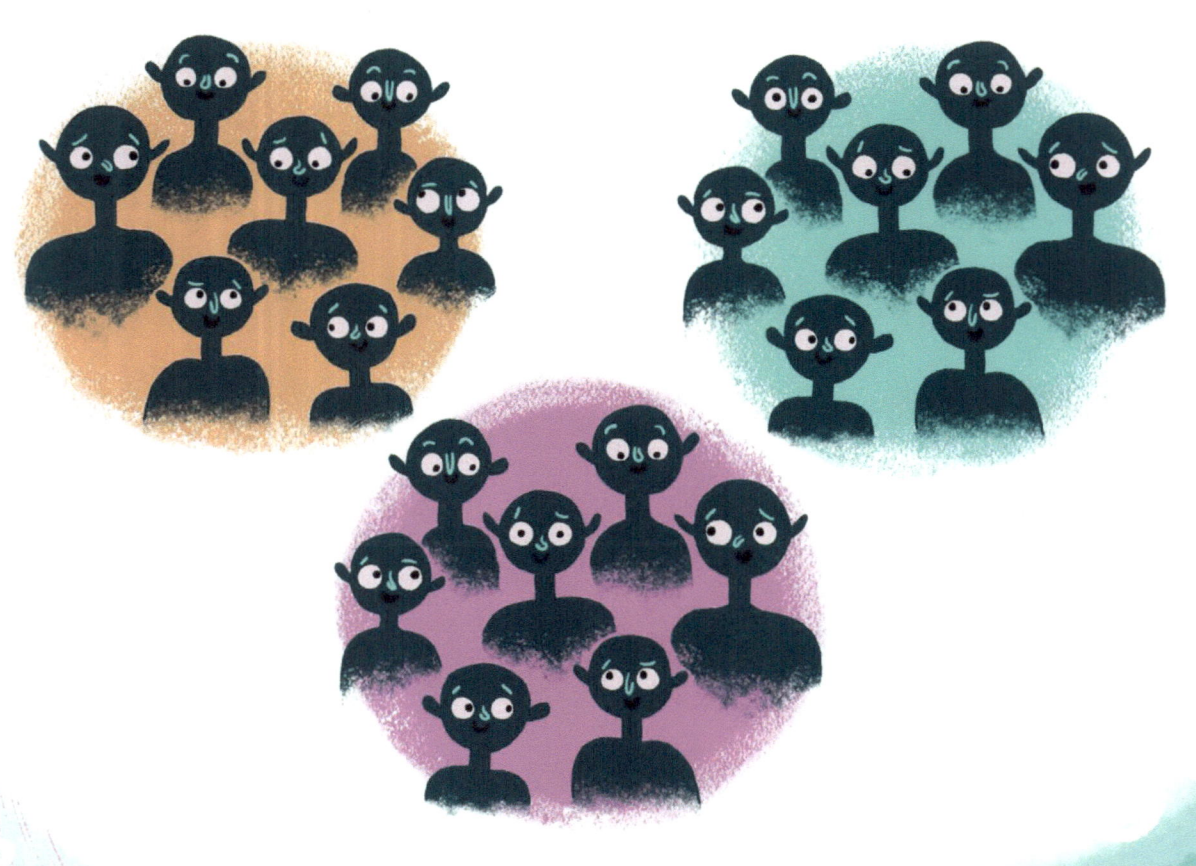

GROUPS CAN INCLUDE PEOPLE WORKING IN A HOSPITAL

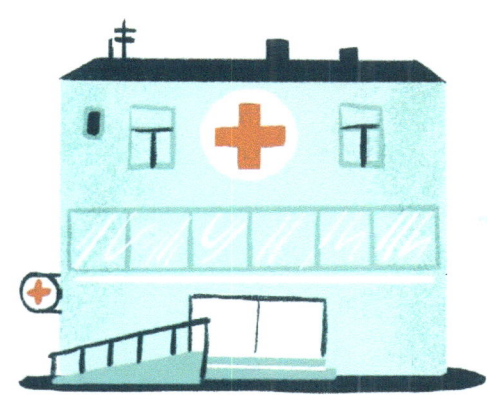
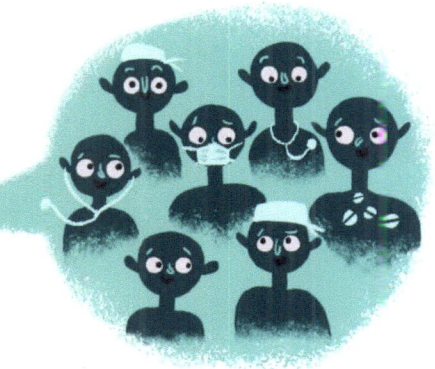
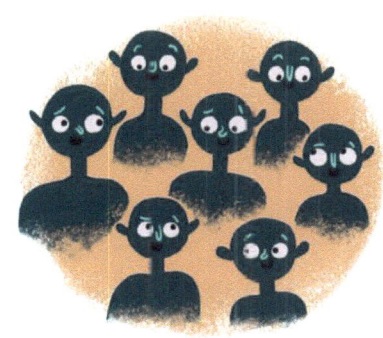
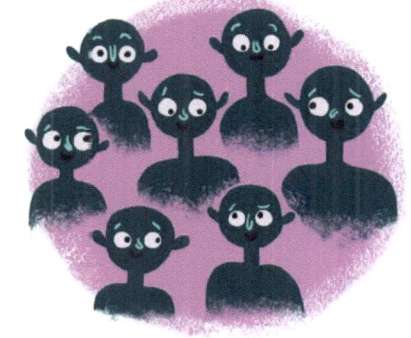

OR PEOPLE WHO LIKE ICE CREAM.

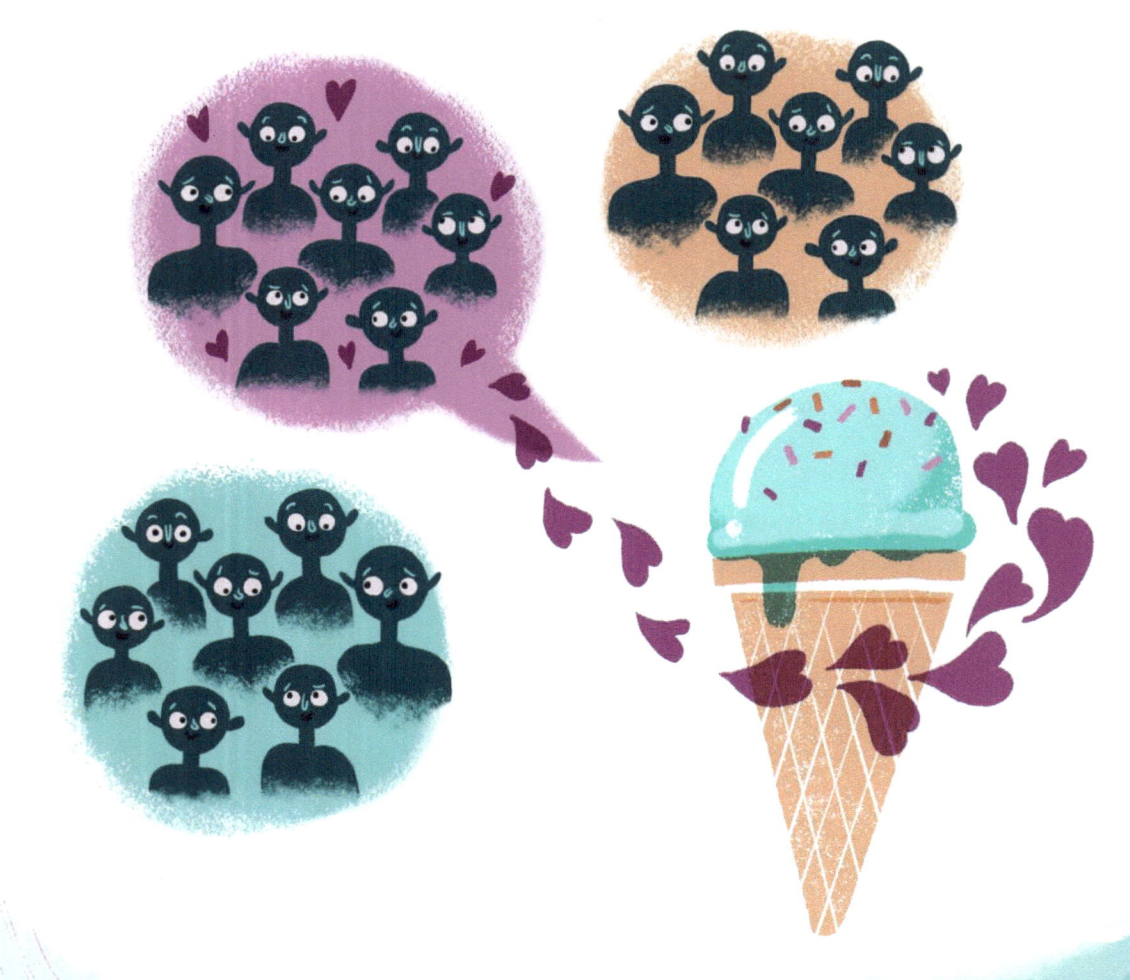

WITHIN EACH GROUP, PEOPLE MAY BECOME SICK.

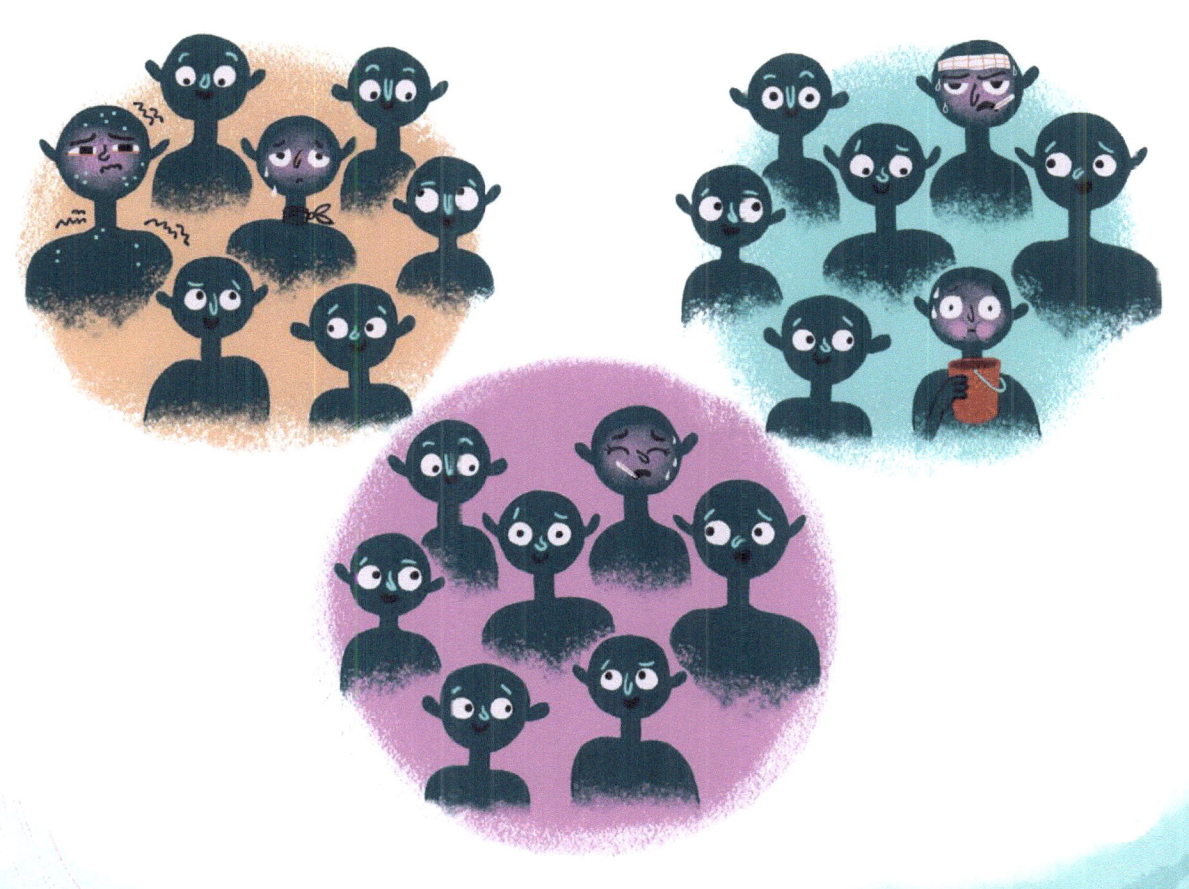

SOME ILLNESSES CAN SPREAD OVER TIME AND AFFECT THE ENTIRE GROUP.

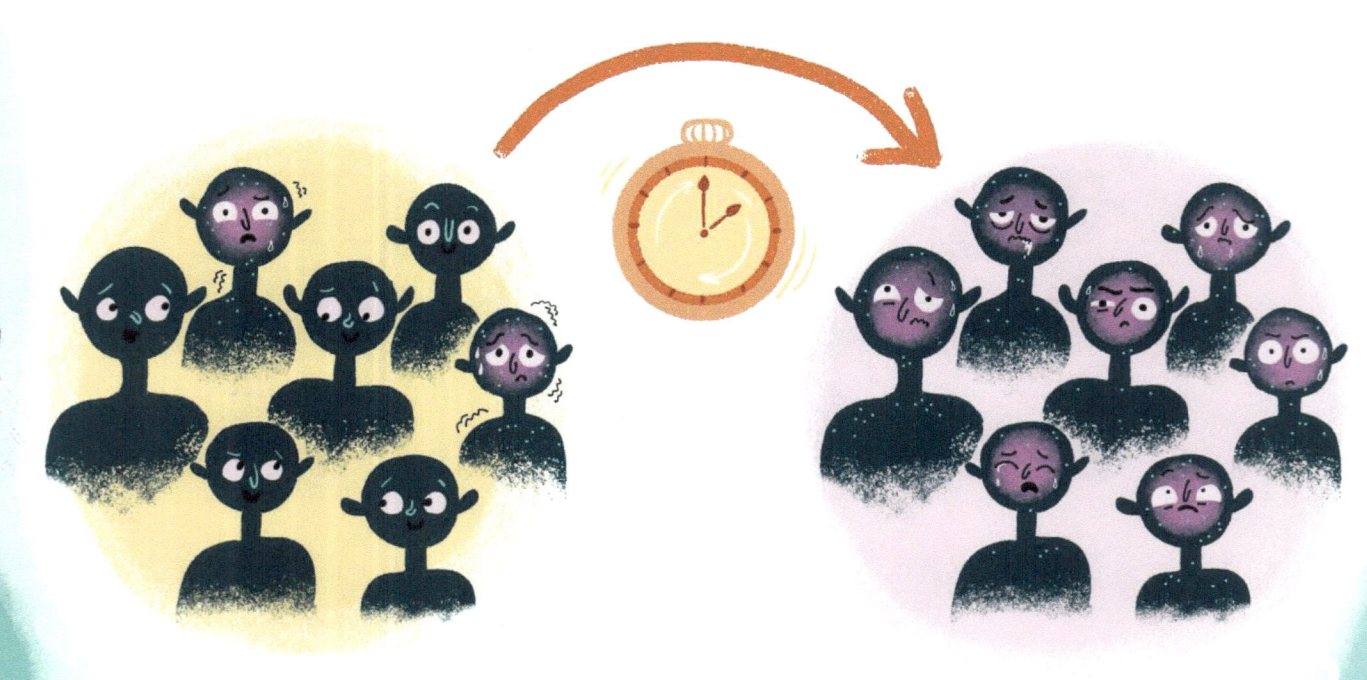

SOME GROUPS ARE **MORE LIKELY** TO BECOME SICK THAN OTHERS.

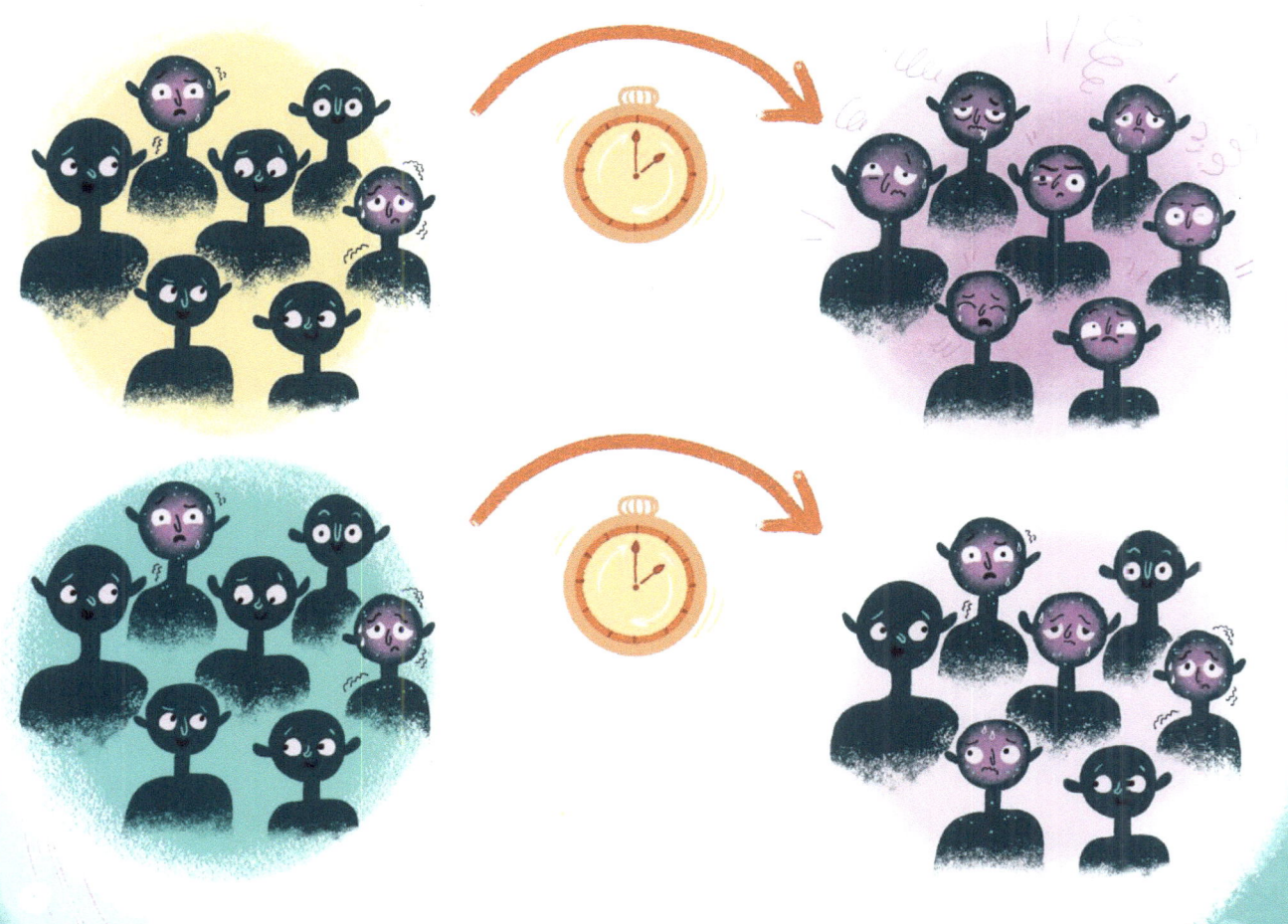

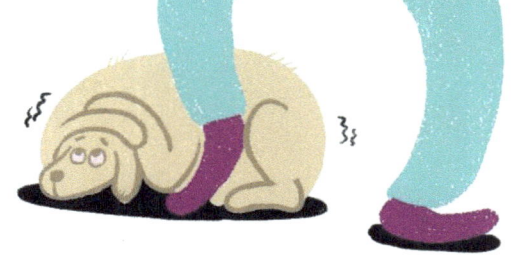

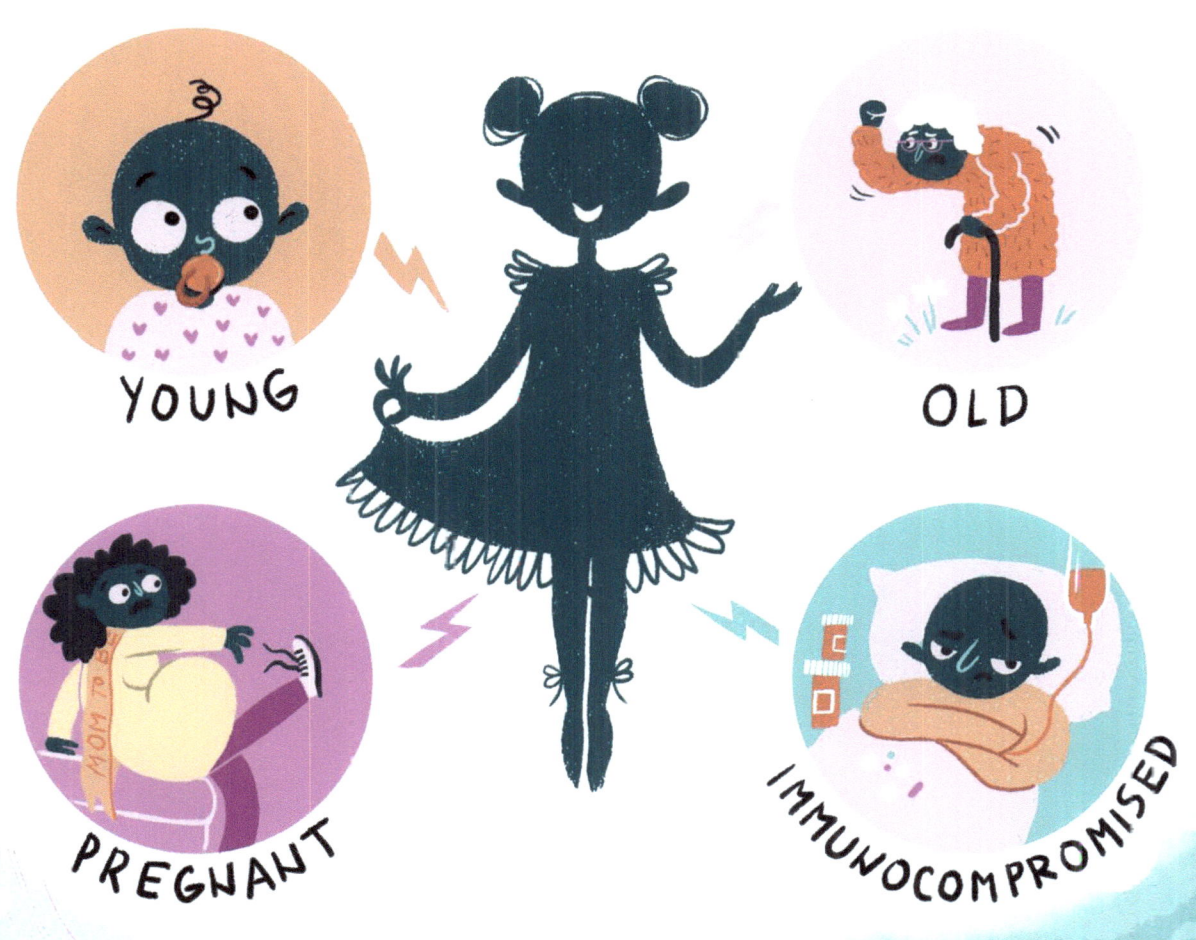

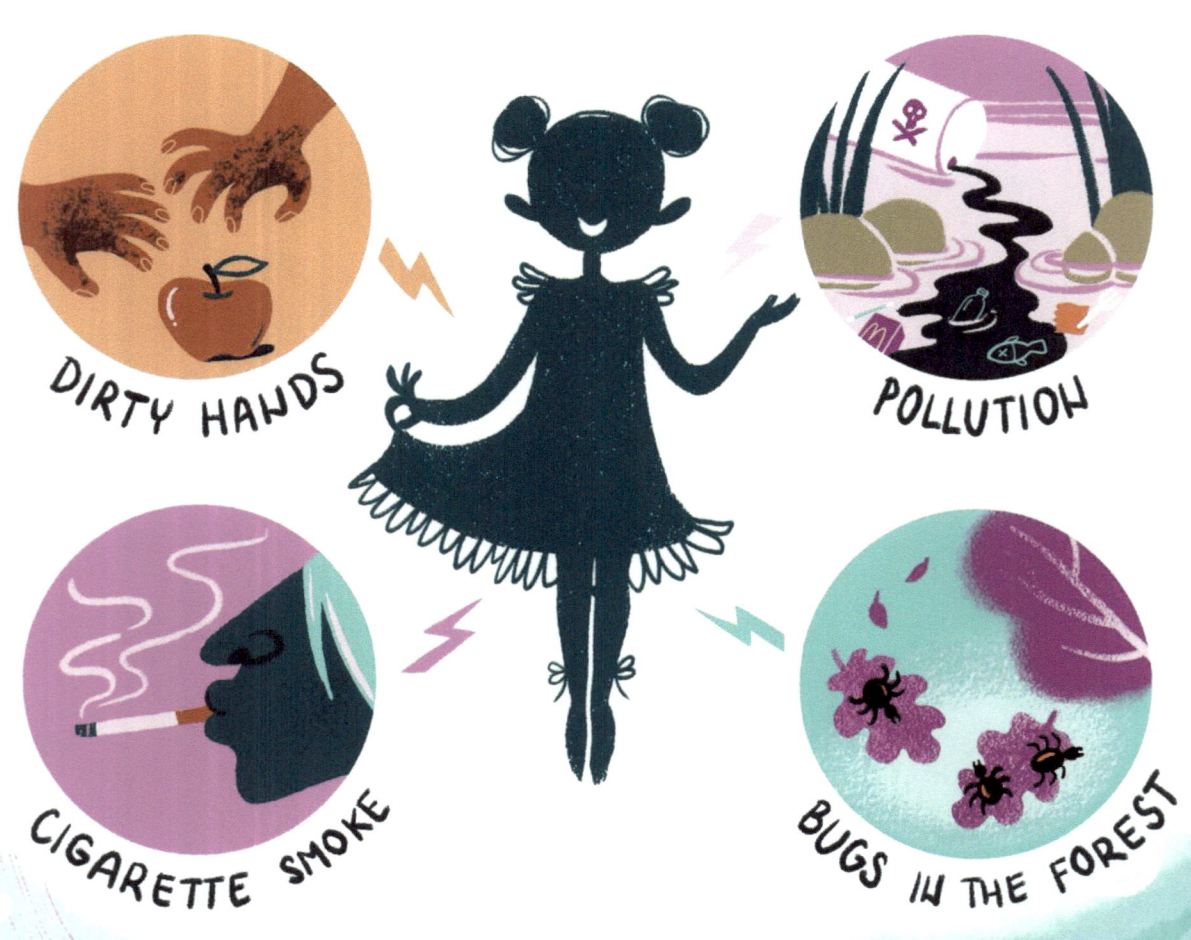

FOR EXAMPLE, OLDER PEOPLE ARE MORE AT RISK OF GETTING SICK.

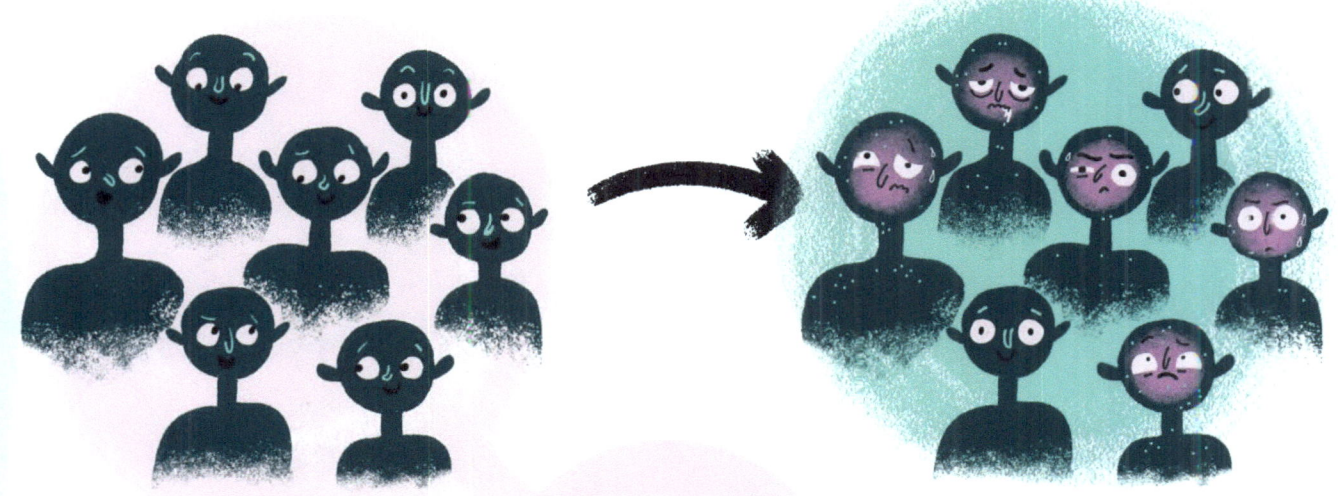

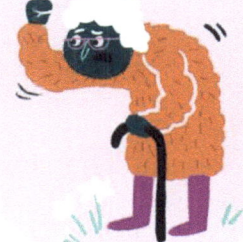

AGE: 85

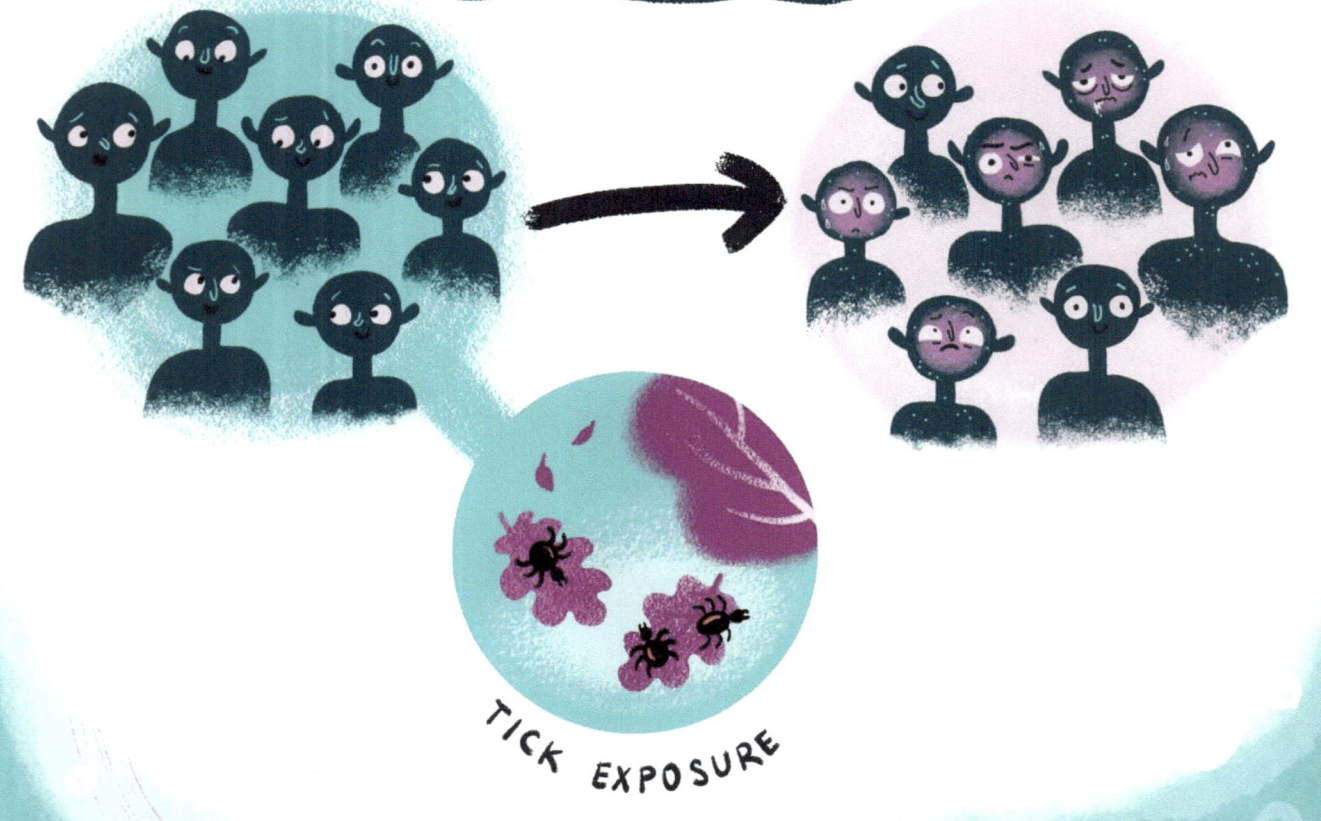

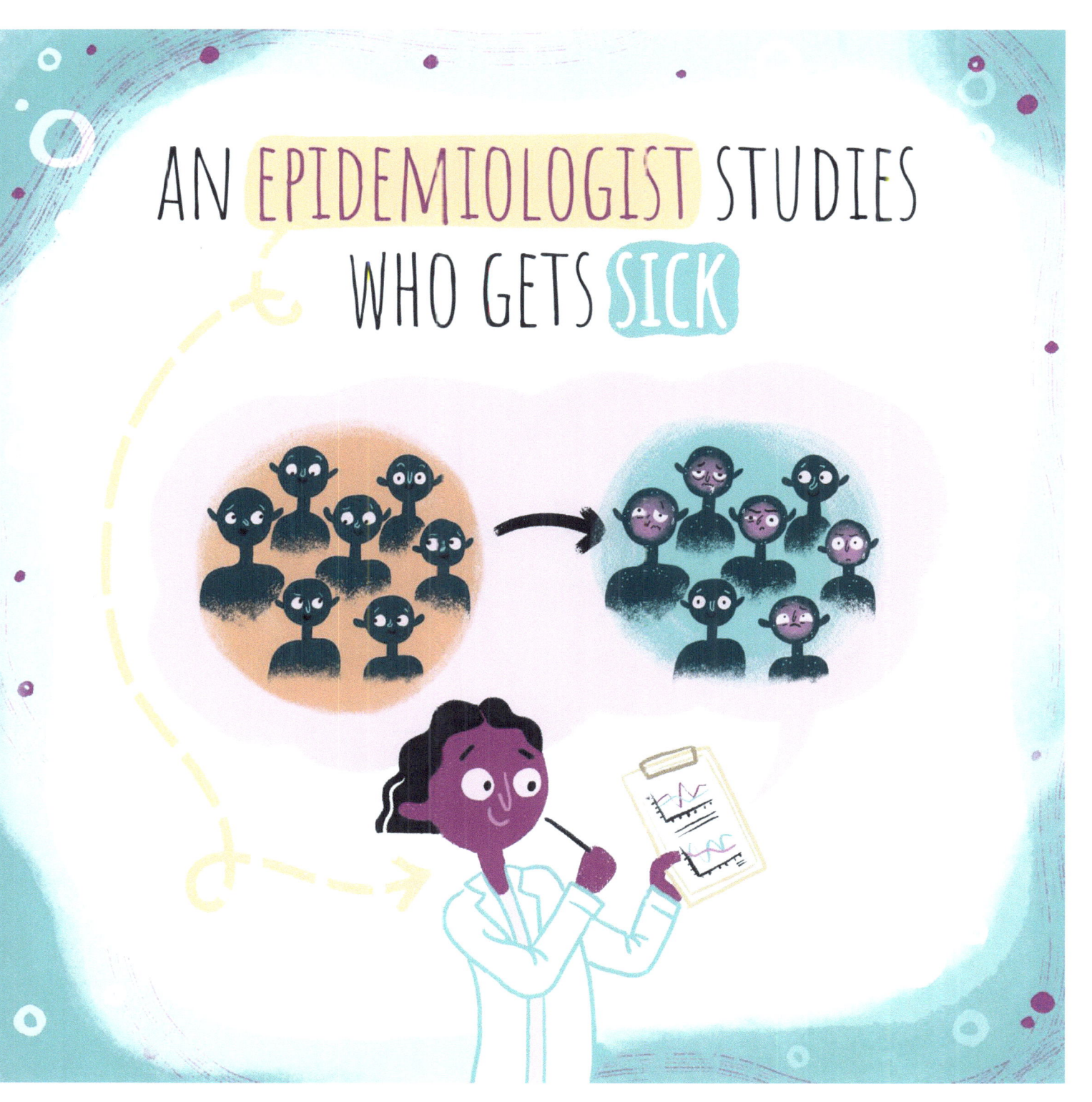

AND HOW RISK FACTORS AFFECT THE HEALTH OF A POPULATION.

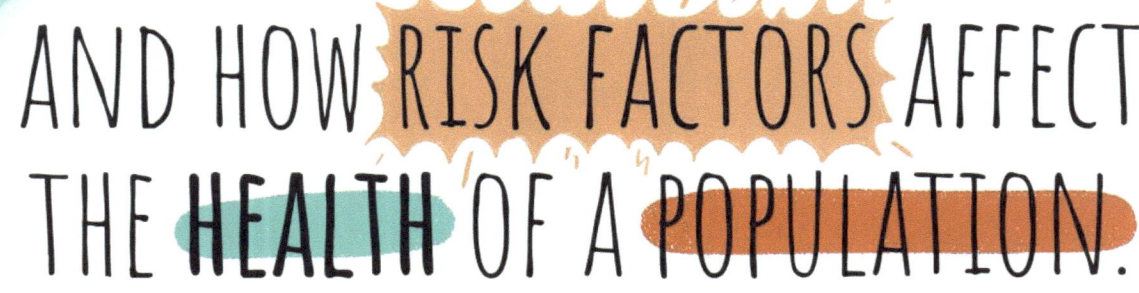

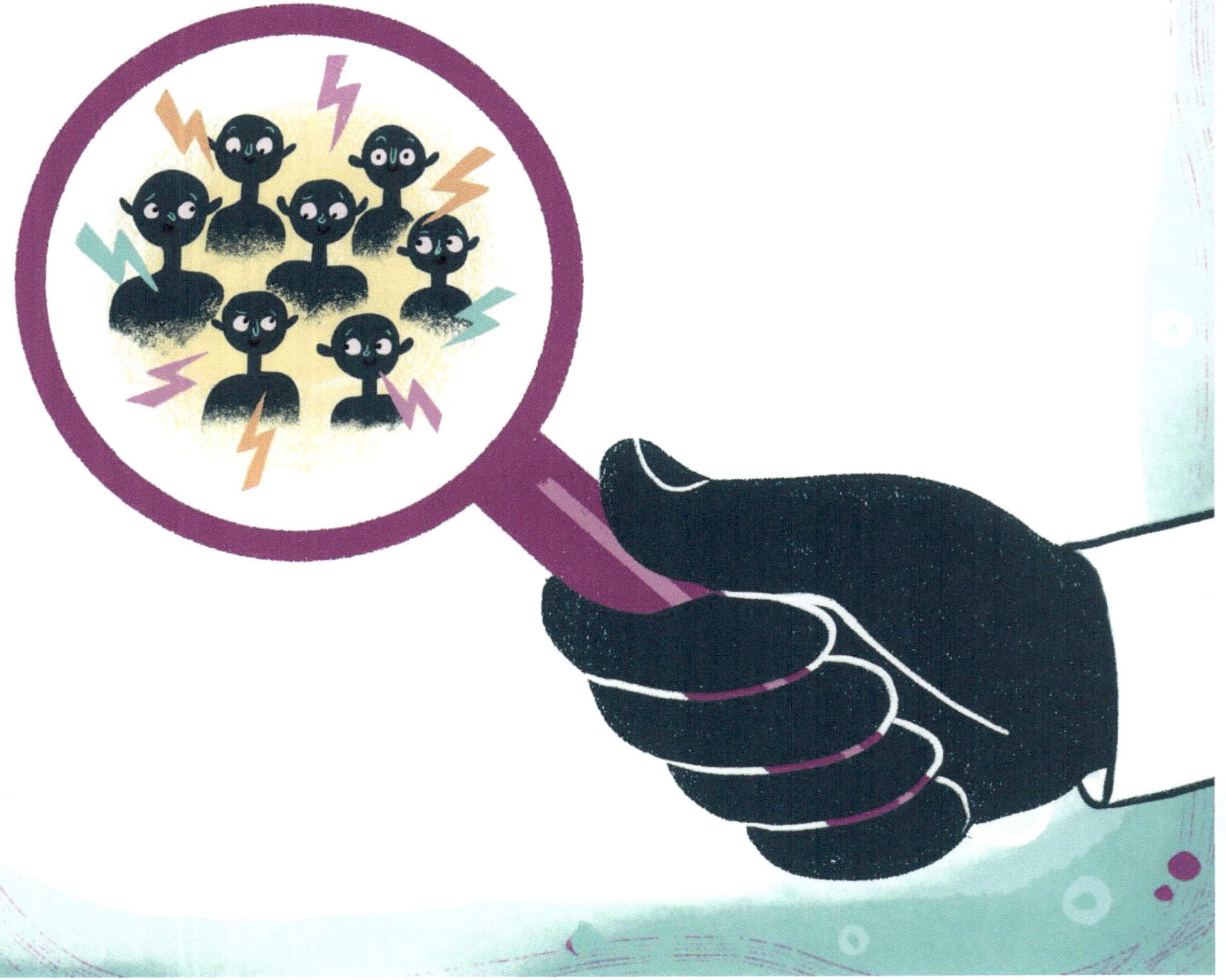

THEY USE THIS KNOWLEGE TO PREVENT AND CONTROL DISEASES.

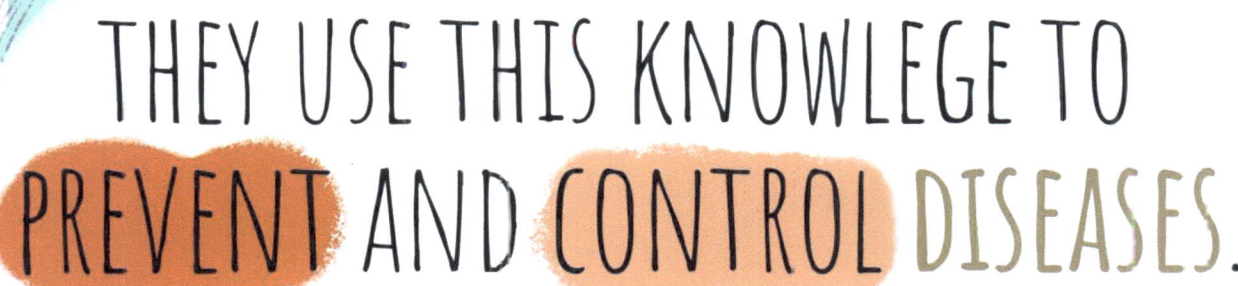

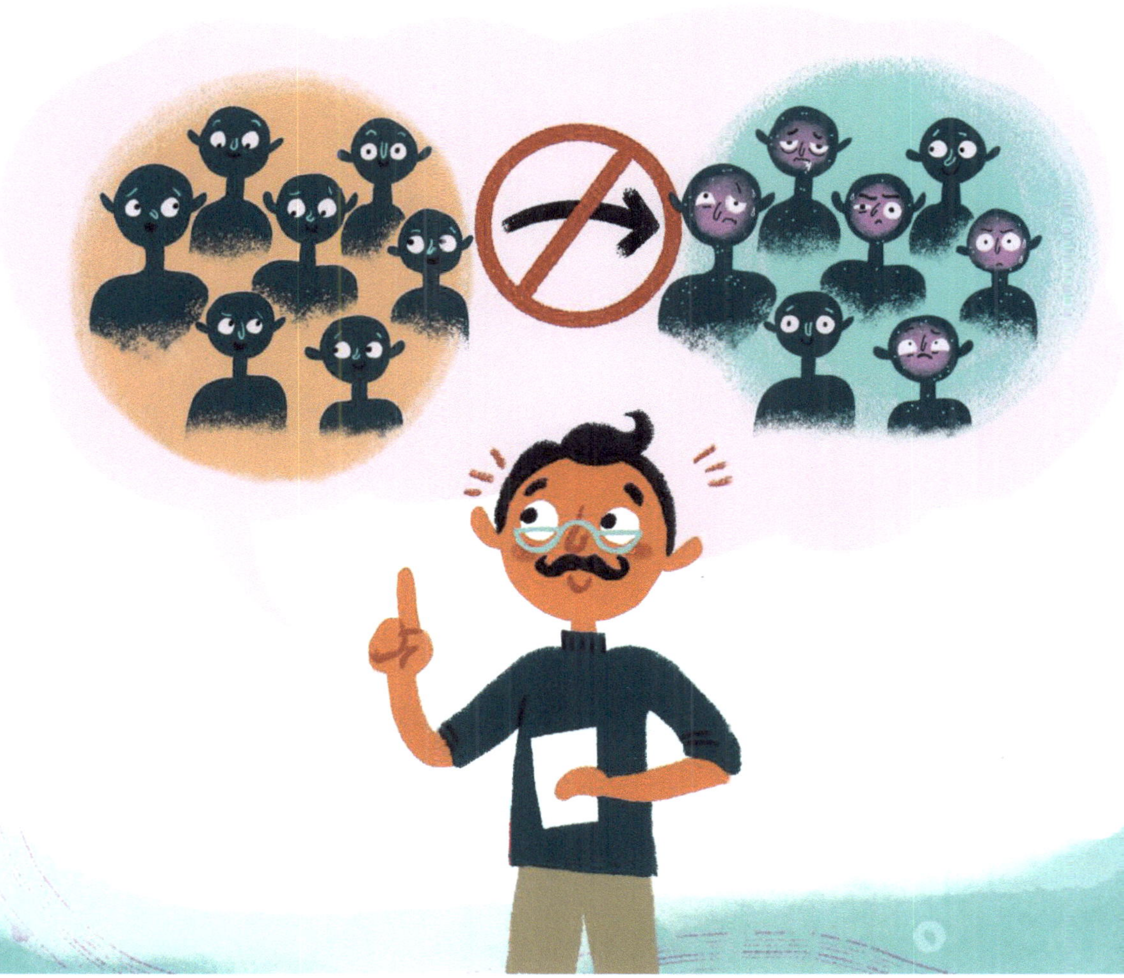

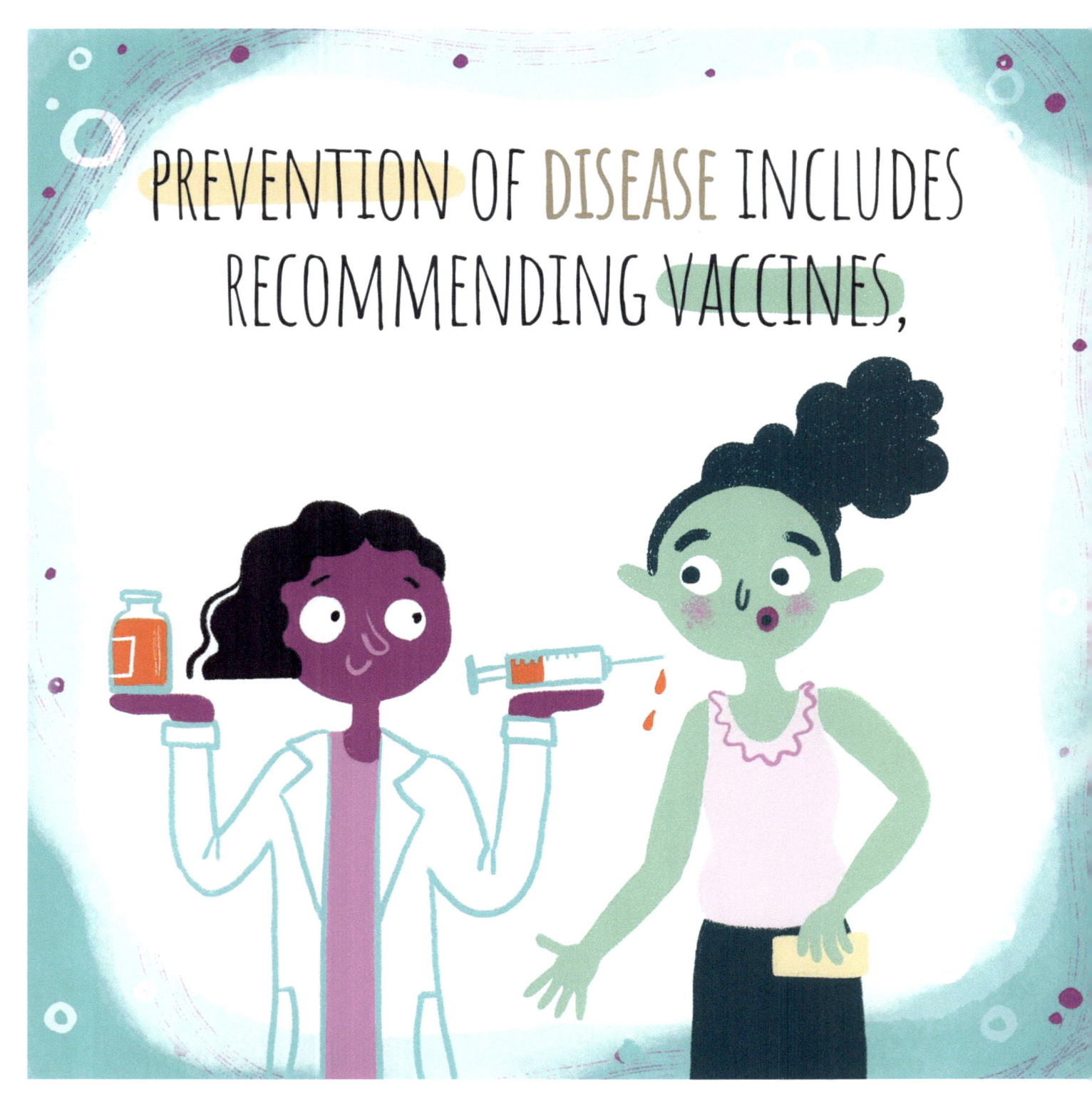

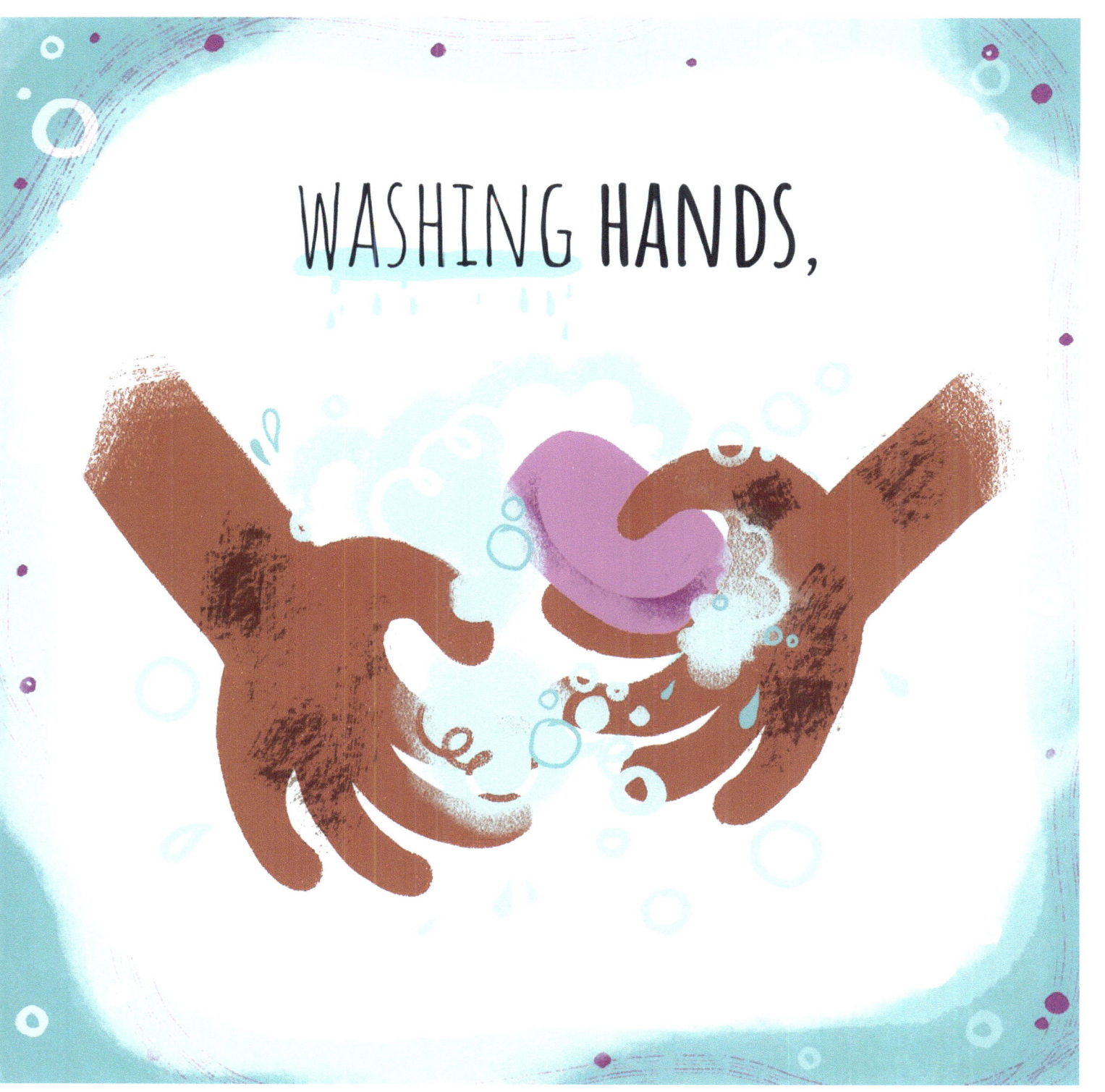

REGULAR DOCTOR CHECK-UPS,

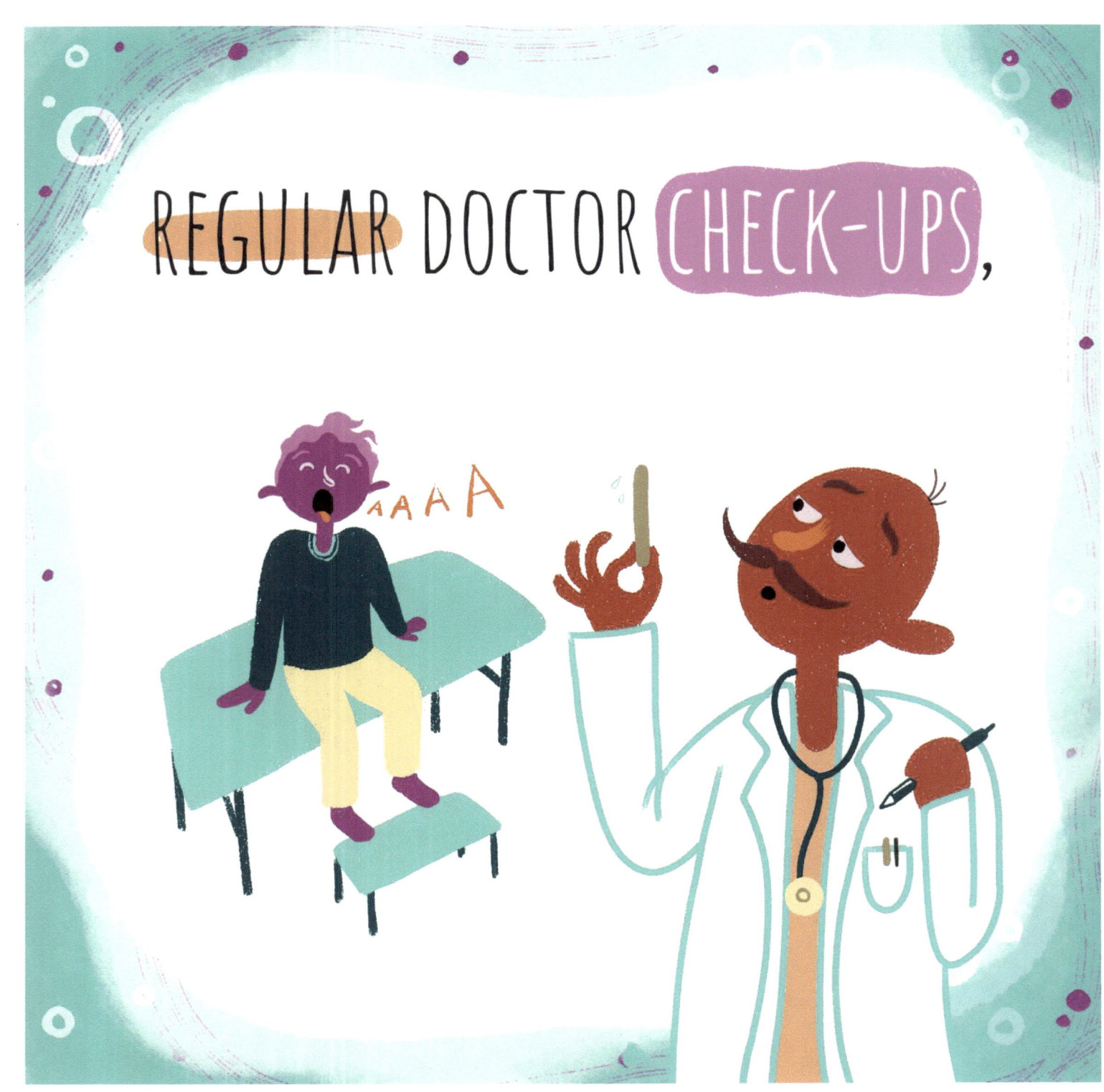

AND PROMOTING HEALTHY ENVIRONMENTS.

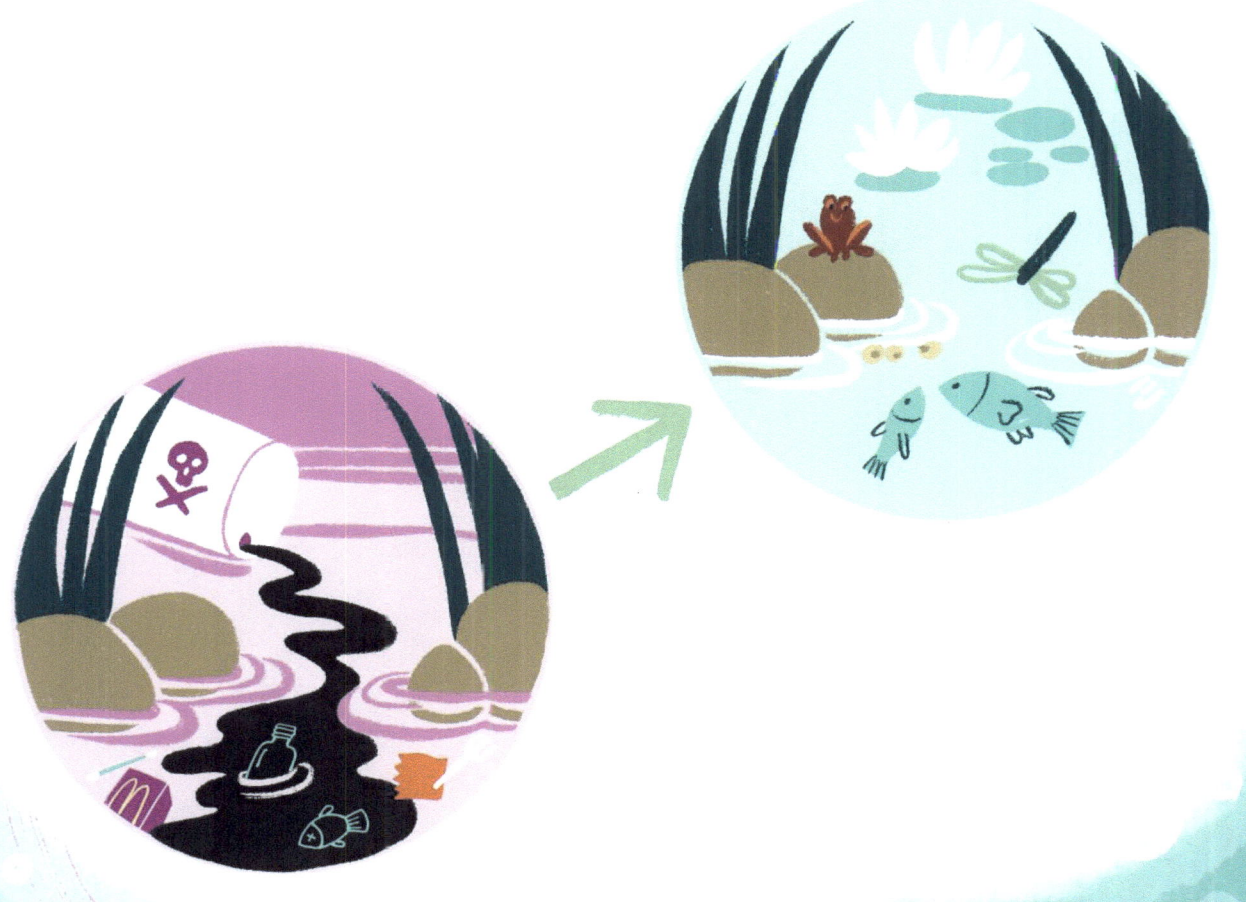

CONTROLLING DISEASE INCLUDES INVESTIGATING OUTBREAKS,

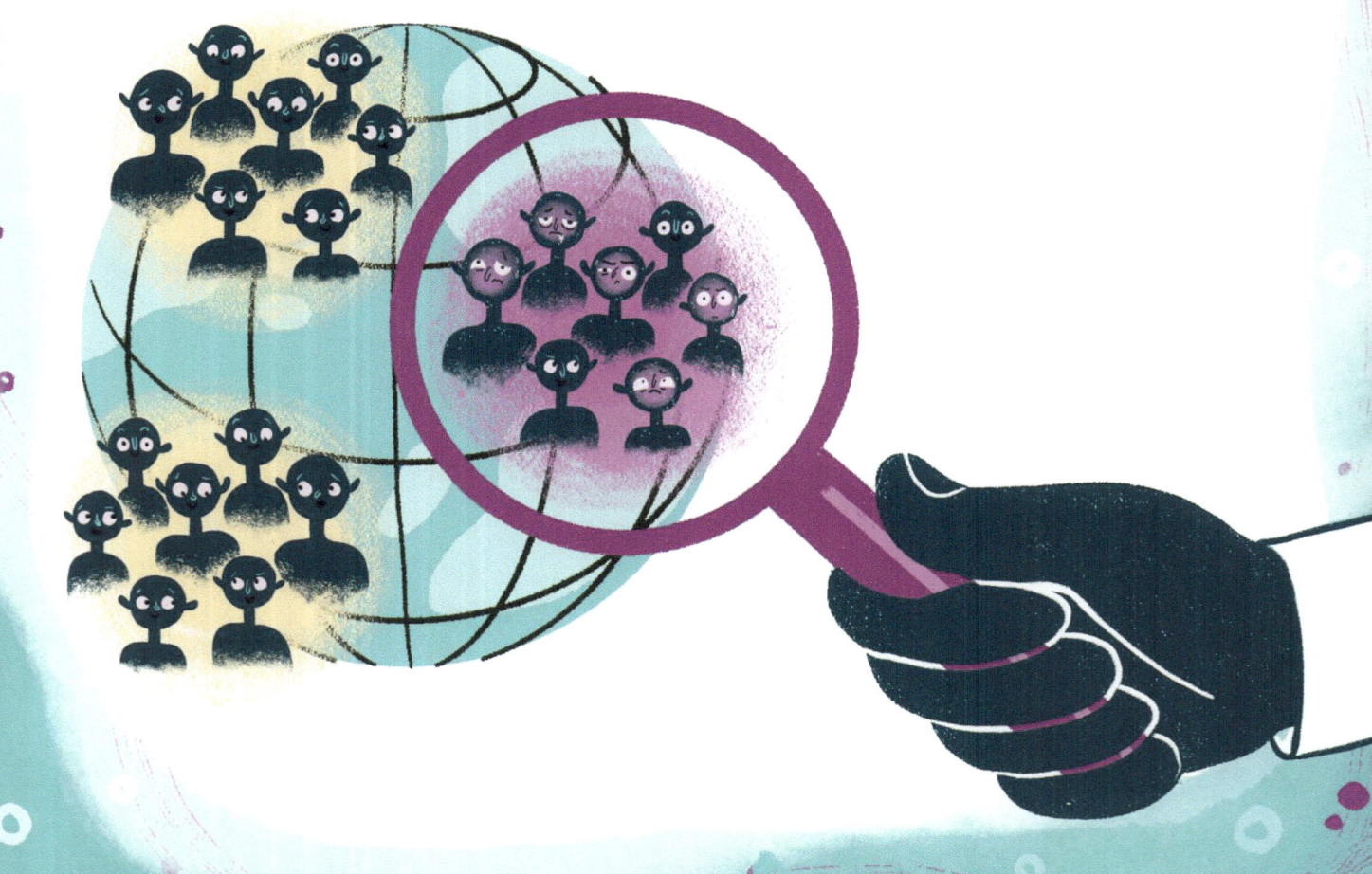

CONTACTING PEOPLE WHO MAY BE AT RISK,

ALL GOOD HERE!

WARNING: RECENT OUTBREAK!

NO WORRIES! ALL HEALTHY!

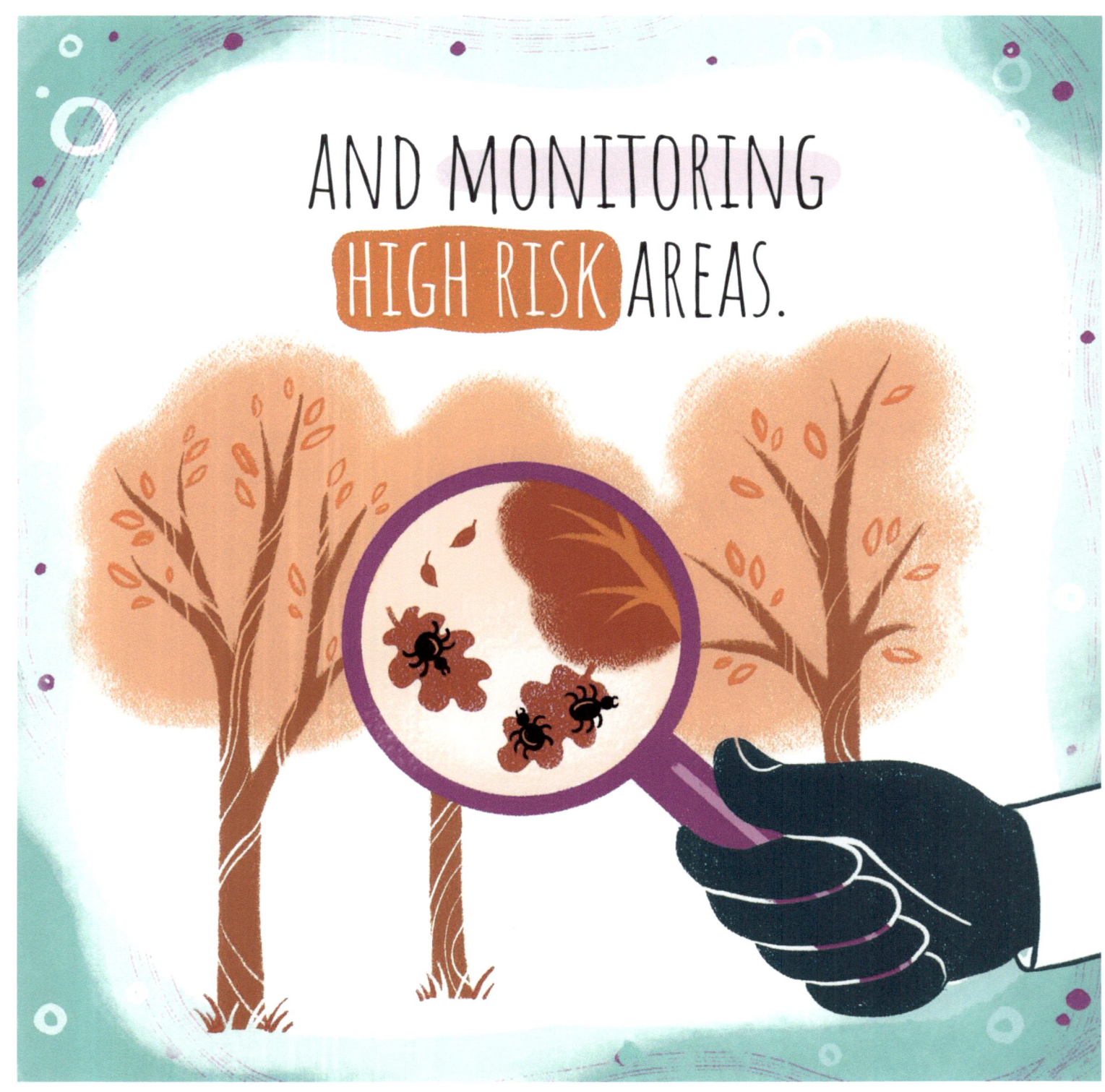

EPIDEMIOLOGISTS COLLECT DATA TO HELP PEOPLE STAY HEALTHY!

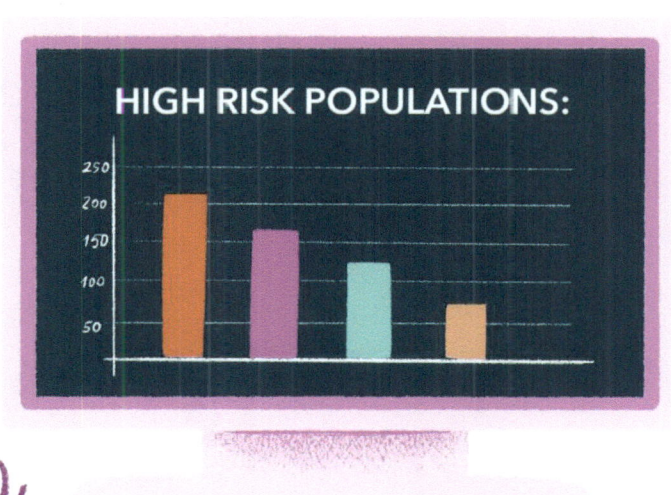
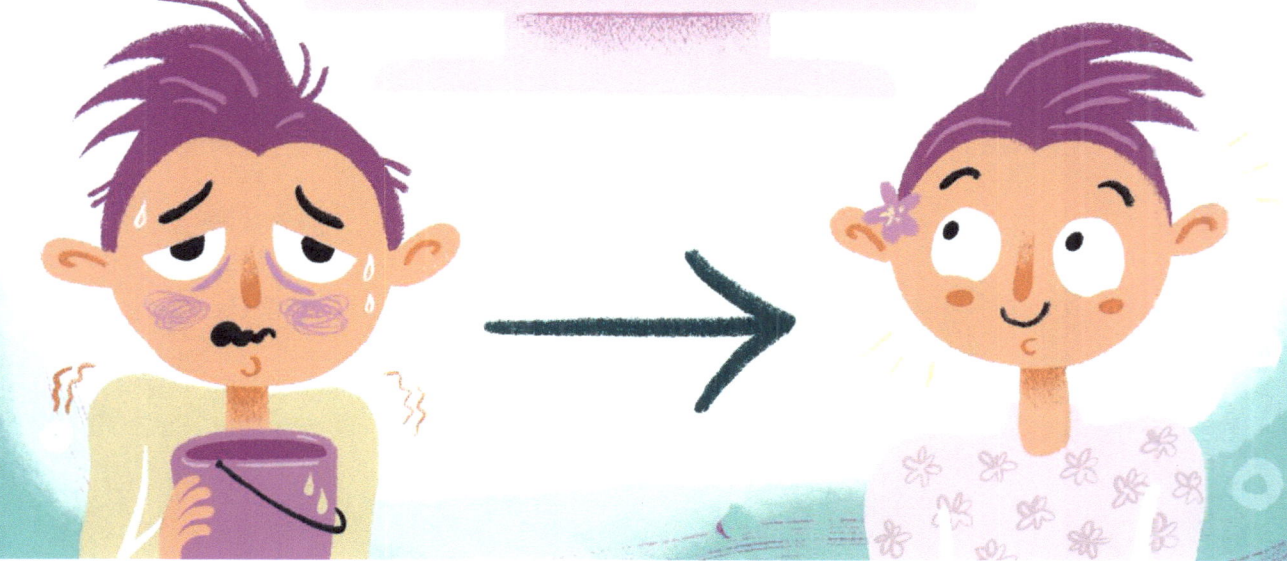

IT'S A GREAT **BIG** WORLD, WITH LOTS OF OPPORTUNITIES...

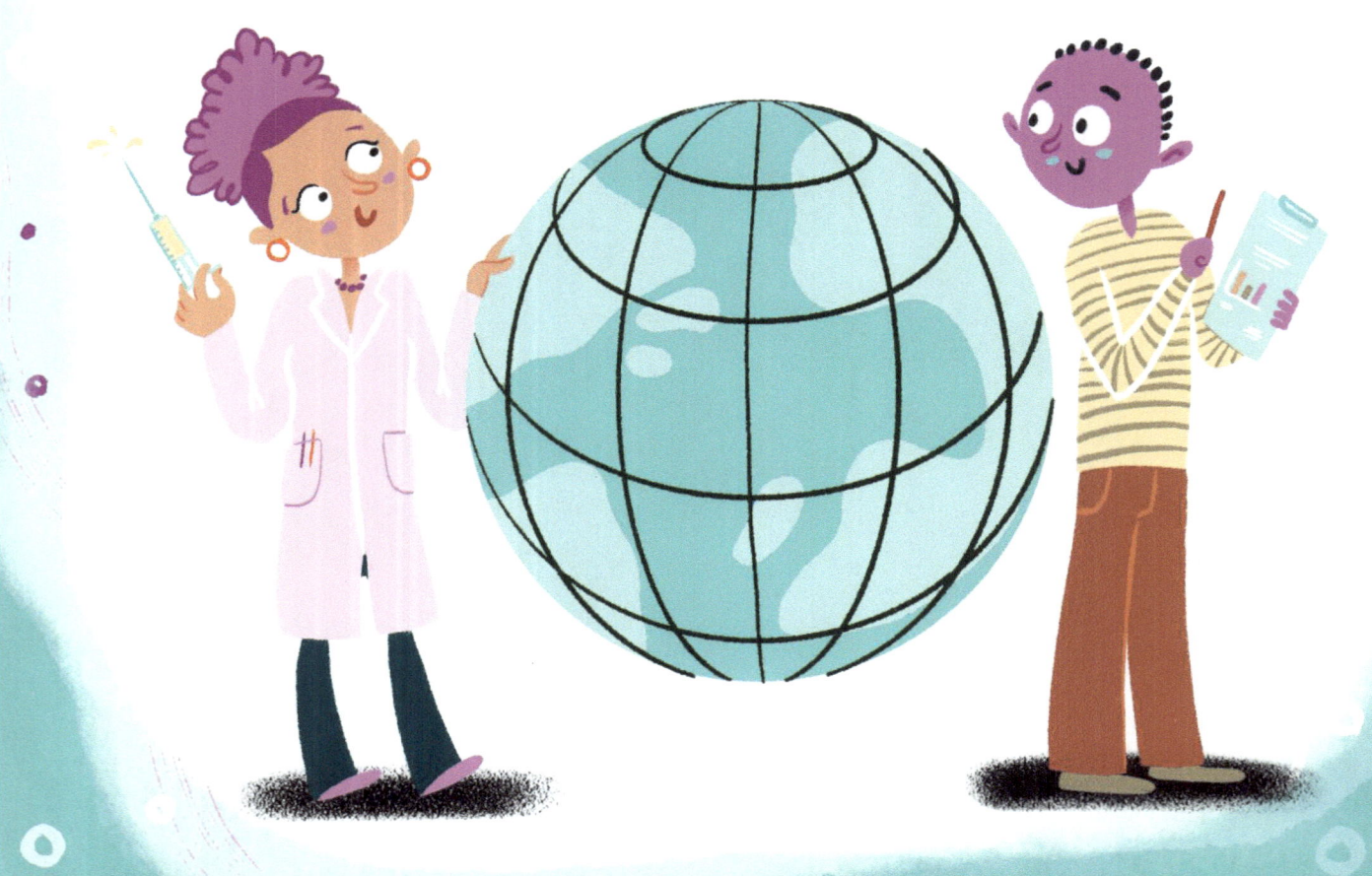

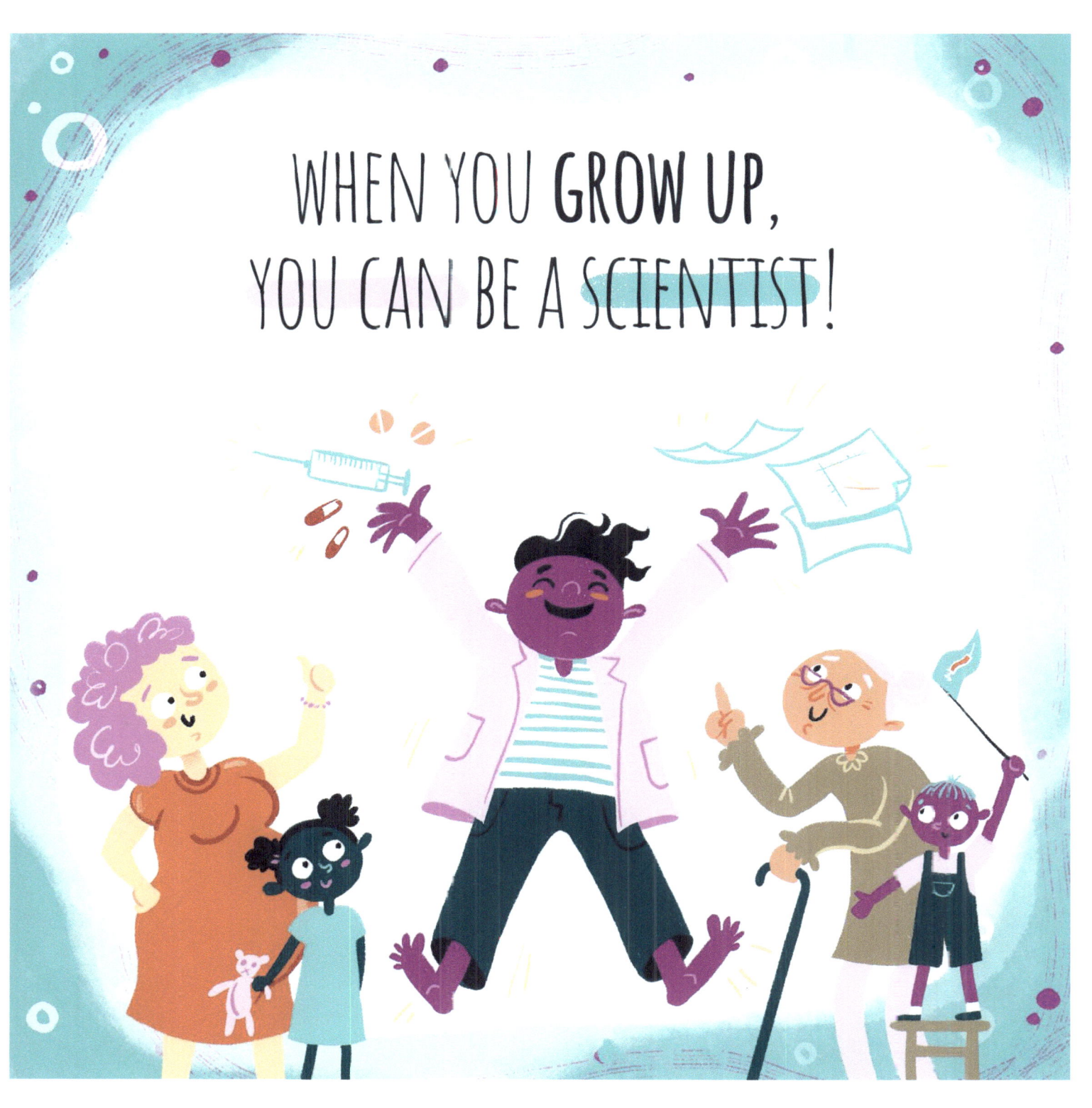